THE CRAIG LEWIS GUIDE TO SURVIVING THE IMPOSSIBLE

Craig Lewis

Better Days Recovery Press

Published by Better Days Recovery Press
survivingtheimpossible@gmail.com
www.sanityisafulltimejob.org

Copy edited by Carolyn McGuire
Additional editing by Emily Ryan and Ali Kat
Production edited by Jonathan Rowland
Cover design by Floh Danku

Contents

Acknowledgments

I give thanks to all who have honored me with their gifts, support and love. I'm alive today thanks to a handful of people who decided that I was worth caring about. I'm alive today because I decided that I was worth caring about. This book exists because you matter; and so do I.

Pets, Punk, and My Pal Craig

I first met Craig at a workshop/speech he gave in Malmö, Sweden in the fall of 2019. I didn't know much about him then, just that he had written a workbook for us peer specialists. A colleague of mine—actually the woman with the most experience in southern Sweden—called him her biggest role model. Since I really admire this woman—her commitment and love of helping others—I was stoked! In walks this tattooed crust punk with pierced ears, and I could tell from the very start just by his aura that he is a kind and loving person; a human that just generates warmth and positive vibes. When he opened his mouth and started telling his story, the room was completely silent.

Well, I'm no spring chicken when it comes to this sort of thing. I've given speeches, held workshops and been in front of crowds more times than I can count, not just as a mental health advocate, but also as a musician. Craig made me feel like a mere rookie. Don't get me wrong, this was a good thing. Actually, it was amazing! I was blown away by his story, how he told it and how he made the whole audience feel included and validated. During the intermission, I walked up and introduced myself. I've been a punk for twenty-nine years, so not only did we connect as survivors but also as punks in our forties. We didn't have much time to talk, but after his speech, we had a very interesting and intense conversation. There were a lot of people that stayed behind and wanted to talk to him, so even if we could've talked for hours about life, concerts, music, and whatever, we had to cut it short, but promised that we'd keep in touch, which we did.

I've been struggling with depression and anxiety since I was five years old. I am a survivor and I've been through hell. I've been through ups and downs and I'm still fighting with my demons every day. Talking to Craig always makes me feel better, even on a good day. Craig always cares, he listens, and he is always dropping little bits of wisdom. He is genuinely himself, and he can't stop that huge heart of his from spreading love. That of course goes both ways. I truly love this guy and when he asked me to write a foreword for his new book, I almost cried. This is an honor and I hope you, the reader, will be helped and empowered on your journey towards recovery. I can't guarantee that this book will solve your problems, but I can guarantee it will get you thinking. It will help you, and if you're looking for proof that surviving the impossible is possible, this is it!

As a peer specialist, I found Craig's first book, *Better Days* to be an invaluable tool in my work and my peers always learn something new during our groups. One of the things I enjoy the most is, when I'm meeting new peers, sporting neck tattoos, and having "PUNX" tattooed across my knuckles, I can say this book is written by a fellow punk from Boston. And in that way, I'm not only helping fellow peers in their recovery, but I can also spread the message that punk is love; it's helping out your fellow man, woman, or however you might identify. When I finally got to read *The Craig Lewis Guide to Surviving the Impossible*, one chapter really stood out to me. It's a subject that I often speak about, and another thing that Craig and I have in common; the love of animals, especially cats. If you're having trouble defining, or feeling worthy of giving or receiving love, what better example is there than the unconditional love from a pet? My old cat, Sonic, was my best friend. He only lived to be ten years old and was sick for nine of those years. I looked after him, and he trusted me to give him medicine for more than half of his life. He saved my life and made me go on when times were at their toughest and I wanted to end it all. Because of Sonic, I'm here today, sharing my message with you.

Hail cats, hail punk, hail life, hail love, and hail Craig!

Christoffer Francke
Malmö, Sweden

Un Buen Amigo

If you've never encountered Craig before, you are in for a pleasant surprise. In this book, you will find an introduction to basic tools for enhancement of your daily life. It's written in an easy-to-read prose/poem style, from Craig's life experiences. Most chapters end with a few provocative thought questions. This is a prelude to his workbook, *Better Days: A Mental Health Recovery Workbook*.

Craig travelled internationally, teaching and providing his methods. His workbook is translated into over a dozen languages. I met Craig through a mutual online friend, and he stayed at my place after giving a workshop in Mexico City.

I am an ex-husband, grad dropout, ex-mental patient, and expat, in that order. A year after my first LSD experience, and months after my first hospitalization (in 1969), I got my real education at the original Woodstock Music Festival. The music was great, but even more important, was the experience of half a million people who were all "brothers and sisters," caring for each other and the earth.

I feel Craig fits right into that mold. I enjoyed his hospitality, staying at his place in Salem, and then got to know him much better in Mexico. His story unfolded to me little by little, as we were together at a punk event, an international hearing voices conference in Boston, and later at a conference in Mexico City.

What's unique about Craig is his ability to convert his extremely difficult past (and sometimes present) life into gold. Without his combination of genius and heart, I doubt that he would have survived, much less been able to find ways to help others. You'll see this in action while reading this book.

Enjoy the fruits of Craig's alchemy by reading and taking his actionable questions to heart. I know this book will improve your life. And share the gold!

Here is his site featuring other texts and products he offers, to uplift the oppressed, and humanity in general.

Don Karp
Morelos, México

Always There; You're Never Alone, From Boston to the Ends of the Earth

I met Craig at "The Pit" in Harvard Square, Cambridge MA, around 1996 or '97. As a young kid from Cape Cod, who truly didn't fit in anywhere. I had a difficult home life where I was not welcome and discovered alcohol as a coping mechanism. Needless to say, alcohol wasn't a good coping mechanism and life did not improve until I was able to come to terms with the pain of my disconnection.

I needed a safe space and safe people in order to thrive. Believe it or not, Craig helped to provide both of those important pieces of recovery for me. He may not even have been aware of how important his presence was in my life back then. We were roommates in Allston, MA. I was never very popular or liked, but that never mattered to Craig. He accepted me and wanted the best for me, and for all of his friends.

I can honestly say, I don't know what might have happened to me without Craig's influence. I was a kid with no home, no parents, and no actual life skills. None of that mattered. Craig was so open about his difficulties and so compassionate towards others, myself included. There were no mistakes that I could make that were too shameful to forgive. Acceptance was the first step towards inclusion and connection. It wasn't until years later, when we had both moved on, that I would fully come to appreciate how fortunate we all are to have Craig as a friend. He works tirelessly for the good of all the people he knows, and he inspires me to do the same.

Craig's traumatic life experiences have been extreme, and he has openly shared his struggles. I am thrilled and inspired by his insatiable drive to help others, despite his own pain. This book is a testament to the amazing resilience of the human heart, against all odds. Written in an easy-to-read style and posing important questions to help us explore our trauma in a way that we can heal, *The Craig Lewis Guide to Surviving the Impossible* is a fantastic tool for compassionate introspection and recovery.

Christina Hungria
Barnstable County, Massachusetts

Punk and Mental Health

My band was invited to do a Mexico tour by the Reacciona family, I traveled along with good friends and met new great people. One of them was Craig. Fifteen years has passed since that tour and while we lost touch for a couple of years, we continue our friendship. Since then, Craig has been a person who has helped me through difficult times and made me realize my potential and helped me cope with depression and anxiety that was haunting me for a long time but hit harder in recent years.

Craig is a survivor, a fighter, and most importantly a friend who, no matter what, will be there.

His story is not for the faint of heart, but he put all that he went through and made a beautiful workbook and traveled the world to help others in need of healing and support—maintaining the DIY ethics and solidarity of the punk scene.

Ismael Flores
Tamaulipas, México

From Survival to Living Life Large!

I've been trying to write this foreword for weeks now. I am a writer at heart and words typically come easily to me, so I haven't understood why this simple foreword should be like herding cats. I think my difficulty has been twofold. One, I want my words to carry heavy weight. My friend Craig has not been supported the way he should have been in life, and that is a grand understatement. I want to convey something more than just a simple, hey Craig's a really good guy and you should read his book.

Second, Craig is not a simple person and explaining him requires words that jump out at you, that paint a picture, that help you understand the depth of personality and character that is my friend Craig Lewis.

To be perfectly honest, the bulk of interactions I have with human beings is somewhere between mildly to profoundly disappointing. My experience with Craig is never like this. Craig has a passion for life, a compassion for all beings, especially those in need, which resonates with me personally and profoundly. This is a man who, although he has been hurt by many humans, will go to the ends of the Earth, risking his own life for another human being in desperate need. I have personally witnessed numerous instances of Craig rescuing an animal or helping rescue a human being from an untenable situation. Yes,

Craig has spent many years in the mental health field. But his behavior goes far beyond what he has chosen as a career. The truth is, that Craig truly believes in love! He believes in love in action and he embodies that love every day. Craig has worked enormously on his own inner growth. He works tirelessly at choosing love over ego, in spite of being on the receiving end of institutional abuse. He is brave and loyal and is committed to living his life on a large scale, capital "L" life. There is nothing lukewarm about this man. And he puts his passion, his personal experience, his whole self into the books he writes to help others.

The international punk culture resonates deeply with Craig and flows naturally from his heart to his actions.

Craig is alive! And if you want to catch some of this contagious life-affirming abundance and largeness, I recommend you join us punks on what could become a crazy beautiful ride of your life toward loving large and living well! Take the first step toward your new life and buy this book!

Karen M. Gagne, MHRT-C
Maine

Introduction

I wrote this book for the purpose of helping myself heal. I wrote this book because I don't subscribe to the idea that because I was hurt as a child, because I was hurt as an adolescent and because I was hurt as an adult, means that the rest of my life has to be of a lower quality than those who haven't experienced these scenarios.

I wrote this book because my heart was shattered before I had the opportunity to know love in a healthy way. I wrote this book because I wasn't shown love, just as my parents were not shown love. I wrote this book because maybe my grandmother's weren't shown love and maybe their mothers weren't shown love.

I wrote this book because I believe that all people are worthy of having an opportunity to heal, to live a good life and to be whoever they were born to be, regardless of what happened to them along the way. I wrote this book because people matter. I wrote this book because I matter. We all deserve to live up to our full potential. I wrote this book because I refuse to stay silent when opening my mouth can help people heal. I wrote this book because I've already paid the consequences for being me.

And who am I? I'm a human being who learned the hard way the difference between being alive and truly living. Thank you for allowing my journey from darkness to light help you shine more brightly as you heal your heart.

This book exists for the purpose of helping make the world a better place.

This book exists for the purpose of helping you truly live.

I am proof that "surviving the impossible" is entirely possible.

If I can survive the impossible, so can you.

Love and Rockets,
Craig "Goyo" Lewis
February 15, 2021
México

A poem titled: "You're Not That Important"

You're not that important, that's the first thing you need to remember.

You think you're important but you're really not.

You really don't matter and you really need to shut up.

Remember you're not that important so get it through your head.

Your feelings don't matter so please stop trying.

You are a problem.

You are a problem.

You are a problem.

You're not that important.

Abuse is as American as apple pie.

Treat people with love, kindness, honor and compassion and watch them heal.

It's as easy as that.

The people who have taught you via their words and actions that you don't matter; they are liars.

Except they're not lying to you; they're lying to themselves.

You are important; read these words and know they are true.

You are not a problem.

Your feelings matter.

You deserve to be treated with dignity.

You deserve to be treated with love and honor and compassion and kindness.

I'm so sorry that you were abused.

"You are not that important" is what they said to me.

It's a direct quote.

To all the people out there who have been told that you deserved to be abused, let this survivor remind you; you have been lied to.

You are important.

You are worthy of dignity, compassion, love and honor. You are worthy of having your story be known and validated.

You really do matter.

I am 100% certain that you matter.

I love you and I love me.

I wrote this poem instead of drinking a glass of bleach.

I like metaphors.

If I can choose to transcend my darkest moments; you can choose to transcend yours.

Love,
Someone who understands the brutality of invalidated pain.

So What?

So What?

You survived abuse.

You survived homelessness.

You survived abandonment.

You survived sexual violation.

You survived physical violence.

You survived manipulation.

You survived deception.

You survived corruption.

You survived emotional abuse.

You survived imprisonment.

You survived legal torture.

You survived discreditment.

You survived humiliation.

You survived devaluation.

You survived unnecessary suffering.

You survived the impossible.

"You're so vain, You Probably Think This Song is About You."

It is; and yet here you are, right here, right now.

In defiance of everything that ever happened to you, you chose to read this book; so let me take this opportunity to share a gem of wisdom that I learned only as a result of surviving everything that you have just read, at one point in my life or another.

Nobody is going to save you; you must save yourself.

No parent, no lover, no girlfriend, no husband, no drug, no doctor, no possession, no car, no nothing.

Nothing will save you from yourself except you.

From the moment you breathed your first breath you have the potential and the capacity to be anything in this universe that you want; for you are made of stardust and you were born for the purpose of showing the world how to love again.

So What? WORKSHEET

1. What is something that's beautiful about you, on the inside, that people who have not been nice to you, would know if they were nice to you? *I was a observant person that can read people n act toward me. I lived in violent home my dad has been in prison when I was even born out of my mom stomach that i can remember. I was raised to be tough not scare of anything that come my way i will react back nice n rude n don't speak period. My moms mom Pastaway as a baby like 5 years as i do see all the time surrounded by alcoholic household, drugs what i seen mom do as i got older enough to know. Never spoke a word n talk i was taught don't say anything or else i get the punishment on regular basis hitting n sexual abuse as well, by men n my trigger watch the 2x. step to me, n not friendly at first give a couple of weeks, i see.*

2. Are you willing to forgive yourself for whatever it is that you did or said, when you were dealing with trauma or an extreme set of circumstances, that impacted your capacity to respond in a grounded, rational and reasonably calm way?

3. Do you know that if you survived any of the things listed in this passage (or other impactful to your life trauma or abuse), that makes you a warrior. It makes you a true survivor warrior or warrioress; it means you have magnificent power within yourself to manifest and to transform yourself into whatever it is you were born to be, no matter what happened to you. Are you willing to accept that you have power and that you can use it to make yourself better?

This is Your Captain Speaking

This is Your Captain Speaking

Have you had enough of being miserable? This is a question I ask myself more often than anyone else is aware.

Does this sound trivial, like a ridiculous question so obviously easy to answer that it may sound foolish to actually ask?

How I would prefer to not feel such dreadful pain upon waking up and considering the facts of my life, for one more day?

Dear Friends,

This is your captain speaking.* This is you, the captain of you, speaking.

Don't you know that you are worth loving?

When you first breathed your first breath; you were as innocent as a kitten or a puppy.

I know you were hurt. I know it was terrible. I know it is unfair.

You do have a choice and as do I; thus, my answer is, yes, I absolutely have had enough of being miserable.

The reality of my life is that I must ask myself this question more often than I would like anyone else to know.

The reality of asking myself this question as often as I do has resulted in these words, thoughts and ideas being shared with you.

*Star Trek

This is Your Captain Speaking WORKSHEET

1.   Have you had enough of being miserable or some other disempowering self-identifying emotion? If the answer is yes; what are you going to do right now in this moment to be better?

2.   Do you know that you are worth loving, no matter what anyone has ever said or done to you and no matter what you have ever said or done to anyone else; including yourself? If you know that you are worth it, please tell the world and make sure that this is what you tell yourself. Questions and answers, questions and answers, questions and answers...

3.   Are you the captain of your ship?

Speak With Your Heart as Words Will Often Fail You

To live with a broken heart is to know that love is real. If you feel pain at the thought or memory of being separated temporarily or permanently, from someone you love; then you get it.

In times of intensity and hurt, please try to remember the little baby you once were, and still are, deep within you; and do right by you.

Your heart is all you got. Protect it. Nurture it. Secure it. Love it.

In this crazy life, too many times, in moments in which I lost myself; my words failed me.

What has been said is done, however, what your heart speaks in this moment, and in every moment forward, is up to you.

Speak With Your Heart as Words Will Often Fail You
WORKSHEET

1.   What would it feel like if every wound in your heart was completely healed?

2.   What is one thing you can do right this minute to reset your mental space to allow for seeing a more beautiful future?

3.   If you could apologize to one person in this world, who would it be and what would you say?

A Self-Love Poem

The most magnificent of all human creatures is you.

If you were taught differently, you were taught wrong.

There is nothing wrong with your spirit that you cannot heal.

If you were told differently you were lied to.

You were born to do good in the world, oh yes you were.

Every fucked-up thing that happened to you happened to teach you the true meaning of love.

I know that's harsh and I know it may hurt and maybe just maybe it is true.

You are a different person than people think you are...

Oh you don't believe me . . . ahhhh yes you do.

I prefer people whose lives burned to the ground.

I prefer the crazies; because we're the best people on Earth.

Did they call you crazy? I hope so. I call you beautiful.

Because if you are or if they said you are or were and you're reading this; then you survived.

You are a miracle.

You are made of steel and yet your heart is pure.

You the person reading this, you are a miracle, do you know that?

I beg of you to pay attention to who you're talking to.

You are a beautiful miracle. Are you listening to me? Are you listening to you?

I don't care what you did or what was done to you; right here right now you are alive, you survived and you are a miracle.

I know what beauty is and it's called love.

Your broken heart can heal; just believe it's true and it becomes true.

If you feel terrible inside it's for a reason.

Something hurt you in your life and you have it within yourself to heal.

And I don't care what they said about you.

They said the same or worse about me.

This is a love song to myself and for anyone else who needs to know that they matter.

I love you.

How To Make Sense of When Someone Tells You That You Need To "Love Yourself" More

For all the hurt kids I know in adult forms. The ones who didn't have the chance to learn love in healthy ways. You are not alone.

We are many. We are so many.

My heart has been shattered countless times.

And I have broken endless hearts.

I don't know how I am alive much of the time. So if you are reading this, and you know what I am talking about, I want you to know that you are great and worthy, and no matter what happened to you, and no matter how you responded; you can cry it out today, tomorrow, next week, or right now.

All I know is that I have no more time to spend being hurt.

My choice is to choose love in every moment, for any other option risks my heart beating its last beat; for humans can only bear so much pain.

We are so many and you are worthy.

I am worthy of being loved.

Say it out loud. "I am worthy of being loved".

We are so many and you are so worthy.

How to Make Sense of When Someone Tells You That You Need To "Love Yourself" More WORKSHEET

1.   When you hear those words "love yourself," what does that mean to you and how does it make you feel?

2.   If you could tell the whole entire world something about you that you think people would appreciate and that they don't know about, what would that be?

3.   What does that word love mean to you and what do you want to do about it?

If You are Having Extreme Thoughts

If you are having extreme thoughts.

It takes one to know one.

It takes one to understand.

It takes understanding that there are reasons why people say and do what they do.

It takes compassion for others and compassion for yourself.

It takes forgiveness.

It takes breathing deeply.

It takes finding safe people to connect with when you need support the most.

It takes knowing that it is "normal" to have extreme thoughts, when you have been deeply hurt and traumatized in life.

It takes stepping back and working hard to make better decisions whenever possible; so you have better outcomes.

It takes forgiving yourself for any freak-outs you may have had and for any interpersonal relationships gone awry, as a result.

It takes deciding that you are worth teaching yourself how to do what many may say is impossible.

It takes doing whatever work you need to do on yourself to strengthen your personal coping skillset to ensure you preserve what you have and allow your life to move forward.

It takes you!

If You are Having Extreme Thoughts WORKSHEET

1.   What is the craziest thing you've ever done and what did you learn from doing it?

2.   If you feel like you are going to go berserk and wreck everything; what are 1–3 things you can do to regain enough balance to be ok? There is no wrong answer.

3.   What are the situations, surroundings and experiences that result in your thinking becoming extreme, and do you believe that if you can answer this question; that you will find deeper insight into what is going on with you and how to make things better?

A Poem of Forgiveness and Healing; For and About My Mama

Dear Mama,

I forgive you for your obsession in harming your child.

I forgive you because I know you are a trauma survivor yourself.

I forgive you because I know your mother abused you.

I forgive you because you were blamed for your reactions to how you were treated.

I forgive you for being so hurt and damaged that you did not learn how to love.

I forgive you for turning that damage on your first-born son.

I forgive you for being scared that your son was brilliant, creative, smart and loving, and that he innocently exposed what was happening behind closed doors.

I forgive you for threatening a psychiatrist with a lawsuit if he didn't give me a diagnosis of schizophrenia and drug me.

I forgive you because you did this to protect yourself.

I forgive you for contributing to me being sexually abused.

I forgive you because I remember every humiliating detail.

I forgive you because I know that deep down inside, you are tortured by things that happened to you before you gave birth to me.

I forgive you for going out of your way to convince anyone and everyone that I was a problem.

I forgive you for being incredibly successful at this because it caused so much more damage than any child should ever be subjected to.

I forgive you for threatening our family members into abandoning me to protect your fragile reality.

I forgive you for your personal involvement in interfering in my relationships with women.

I forgive you for abandoning me in 2017, when I trusted you for the last time.

I forgive you for threatening me with an ultimatum that if I didn't stop talking about what happened to me as a child, in your home, that I would no longer have a family.

I forgive you for seeing that threat through and making it a reality.

I forgive you because I refuse to allow what happened to you continue to harm me.

I forgive you because the cycle of abuse ends here and now with me.

I forgive you because you cannot forgive yourself.

I forgive you because you turned down my offer of unconditional reconciliation and public forgiveness simply so I can know what it felt like to have a mother and be loved.

I forgive you because all I wanted was to have my mother tell the world that I was a good, smart, dignified, and honorable man; and you weren't capable of doing this.

I forgive you because you'll be gone soon.

I forgive myself because I'm not sure that when that happens, if my tears will be of sadness or of relief.

For anyone reading this, I ask you to please not allow my mother's abusiveness to be in vain.

Sometimes we need to be destroyed to be properly built.

My mother nearly destroyed me and here I am.

I share with the whole world; the power of my love; the power of my joy; the power of my gratitude; the power of my forgiveness and the power of my honor.

I chose to be happy as an act of defiance and love.

I'm the author of my life and you are the author of your life.

Believe in miracles; because the words you just read are written by one.

How to Forgive the Unforgivable (Because You Deserve Peace)

I grew up in a home that was very comfortable. We always had food, nice clothes, nice cars, we went on vacations, out to eat; I never had to worry about material and tangible needs.

Sadly, I don't recall being loved.

There was lots of talk about "love" but love was just a word.

Love, I was taught, operated on a Quid Pro Quo system.

Do you know what I am talking about?

If you did the right things, according to the hand that feeds; you are fed well.

What if doing the right things for you meant that your decisions were unacceptable for someone else?

What if there were repercussions for simply doing the right thing . . . ?

The abused child is taught confusion.

The adult they become cannot always be sure if they have healed and transcended this confusion or if it became part of who they are?

The lack of intention in the survivor's reaction, and the vile explanation behind the behavior; often, so it seems, are lost, in favor of punishment, abandonment and betrayal.

If you would not yell at a three-year old who had an "accident," why scream at the adult who was taught the ways of the world via abuse?

If you become this adult, and the world scorns, degrades and forcibly detaches you; then you will learn the hard way that forgiving the unforgivable may possibly be your gateway to peace.

How to Forgive the Unforgivable (Because You Deserve Peace) WORKSHEET

1. I bet there is something upsetting you that you've never been validated for. After reading the passage above, what are you going to do today to improve your life?

2. For what reason do you think that you survived everything that's ever happened to you?

3. My definition of love is _____?

To Heal from How Others Have Hurt You May Require You First Forgiving Yourself

Forgiving yourself for responding the way you did, because of what happened to you may be the hardest thing you will do on your journey for healing, recovery and in living a better life.

Every single person on this planet is fucked up.

This is the truth that most people don't want to admit.

My name is Craig Lewis and I have nothing to lose, so as you are reading this book that was authored, based on my own experience of learning how to survive and transcend the impossible; I refuse to give you anything less than 100% purity from the well of my soul.

This book in part is my letter of accountability to those who have harmed me throughout my life.

I spent a lot of time trusting other people, believing that their word was bond and that they would help me. It is easy, so many think, to throw the baby out with the bathwater and not give credit where credit is due. Well, whether you view all your experiences as unfortunate or fortunate, you still need to deal with what happened.

This is one requirement for healing that I am currently learning how to do. I need to be successful and the only guarantee that I can make to myself, is that I will always do my very best to love myself and heal, so I can live the life I was born to live; no matter what.

To Heal from How Others Have Hurt You May Require You First Forgiving Yourself WORKSHEET

1. If you can write a list of all the people who hurt you, you can also write a list of all the people who helped you. Even if the only name you write is your own; that's good enough.

2. Deep down inside, we're all screwed up. Do you believe that you have the power to radically transform yourself, and what's one thing you can do today to rise up and be the person you were born to be?

3. The author of this book is an abandoned child; it's brutal. Nevertheless, if I could get myself together enough to make this book a reality; then I am all the proof you need to know that surviving the impossible is absolutely possible. I have to forgive myself several times a day to be okay. What do you have to do to be okay?

If Your Animal Companion Loves You Unconditionally

If your animal companion loves you unconditionally, maybe they see the true beauty that exists within you.

I will always always always cherish the love of my sweet little boy, Max the Cat.

No matter where on this Earth he is, breathing or resting in peace; he loves me and I know it.

Saying goodbye to Max the Cat was one of the hardest and most painful experiences of my life.

I feel that I abandoned my child, my rescued best friend to whom I dedicated myself to caring for for the rest of his life.

How blessed are we all to know that months after he returned to the street, after his foster mother who loved Max as much as I did was displaced and has now passed away; that he is now adopted by a loving family; once again, and he is now safe and cared for for the rest of his life.

I call him my "Sweet Beast," and he is my best friend.

Through thick and thin; this 28-toed furry creature loved me; in defiance of my many hard times, my ups and downs and several instances of absolute chaos and crazy.

It has been a long time since I felt the warmth of Max the Cat, however, I will never forget the power of his love for me.

If he loves me, no matter how rough or terrible things were with me; then I must be worth it, right?

People often say "animals know," so trust in your four-legger, your feathered friend, your amphibious roommate and even your aquatic amiga.

So perhaps, on those days, when it is hard to imagine that tomorrow could ever come, like I felt a mere three days ago, perhaps remember that if you have ever been loved unconditionally by your animal companion; maybe they know what they are talking about.

If Your Animal Companion Loves You Unconditionally
WORKSHEET

1.   What is your most beautiful memory or thought of an animal companion that once was or currently is in your life?

2.   Do you believe that your animal companion views you as the most beautiful, perfect, special and wonderful creature in their life?

3.   If your animal companion said to you, in words, how much they love you; what would those words be?

A Special Crazy

As many are aware, I do believe in miracles because I am the living proof.

But you are feeling upset, you say?

Si, my brain plays tricks on me when _____ happens.

Sometimes I think I really am crazy.

The truth is; I am.

I'm just a special sort of crazy; a better crazy; a beautiful crazy.

It is a good thing.

You can embrace yourself too; you are cool.

With the cicada symphony as my bedtime soundtrack; I trust in all things beautiful and true.

Do you?

A Special Crazy WORKSHEET

1.   What is a miracle and name one miracle that you have experienced?

2.   Do you believe that your thoughts result in the feelings you feel?

3.   What does it mean to have your brain play tricks on you and what do you think you can do about it?

Harm Reduction For Complex Post Traumatic Stress Disorder Survivors

If you're a person like me, then you know a thing or two about gooooooiiining craaaaaaazyeee.

If you're a person like me, then you view the world and people in a very different way.

If you're a person like me, then you know about unnecessary loss.

If you're a person like me, then you experience how people treat you in ways that the rest of society often cannot understand or comprehend or empathize or appreciate.

If you're a person like me, you may have already considered ending your life today, as part of your daily life experience, and yet since you're reading this you are here now. Thank the Universe.

If you're a person like me, then you know that most people who know you have experienced you gooooooiiining craaaaaaazyeee. They don't understand that you are overflowing with so much love that anything that diminishes your true beauty feels like a death blow.

Because they don't understand and cannot understand; It is easier for them to walk away.

If you're a person like me, then you know how easy it is to resolve the things that get you in trouble. If you're a person like me, then you know how hard it is to get anyone to listen to you and actually help you resolve the things that get you in trouble.

Today is Friday, August 30th, 2019. I desperately needed help and I could not get it. It is common for me that minor issues erupt into major crises, that are avoidable. So I helped myself.

In an act of self-love while choosing to live in the moment; I chose to do something that is harmful and has consequences. Indeed, I chose life. I chose to celebrate and nourish the natural beauty that exists within my heart. Yes, I absolutely chose to do something that is harmful and has consequences; and my choice allowed my blossoming to continue.

I knowingly overdrafted my bank account to make sure I had safe housing, food and basic needs met. I knew that if I had my needs met, I could do everything else that I needed to do.

It is interesting, that the difference between me being "mentally well" and some bastardized version of mental health, in diagnostic word form, is often so basic; shelter, food, water, safety, clothing, employment, the most basic and necessary levels of Maslow's hierarchy of needs.

It is amazing to be grateful for being misunderstood—It forced me to save myself, and I did!

Harm Reduction For Complex Post Traumatic Stress Disorder Survivors WORKSHEET

1.   If you're a person like me; then you understand what it means to:

2.   Here is something about you, that if others understood; they may treat you much better.

3.   No matter what anyone says, thinks or does, what are three things that are beautiful and special about you?

A Problem is a Solution in the Making

If I sound like I'm a broken record, it's because I sound like I'm a broken record.

One thing that not everyone reading this may be informed on is that music, back in my day, was listened to on a record player.

To use the phrase "like a broken record," is speaking in an idiom.

That's why it's so important that we consider the magnitude of the weight and power that our words carry.

So, what does this have to do with the title of this passage?

When I say a problem is a solution in the making, do you see how easy it is to change everything with one single thought?

This is your job.

You are your job.

You can either make your life better or make it not better.

It doesn't matter if you messed up 18 times today, and it's only 4:17 PM; because 19's a charm.

A Problem is a Solution in the Making WORKSHEET

1. Because the author of this guide is a Punk Rocker, and a music lover, making a reference to vinyl records; what is the wildest and/or most impactful or life-changing song or band or album for you in your life? Why?

2. Do you know what "ego" is and how it affects your decision-making, perception and how you view yourself, others and the world? I recommend looking up the definition of "ego" and figuring this out yourself.

3. People who know me well know that I don't like to use the word "problem." I usually spell it out, because I don't believe that such a thing exists. What is one life-improving lesson you have learned as a result of surviving your most painful struggles?

Happiness is an Illusion, or is it?

When you say that you're happy what does that mean?

Are you happy because the emotion you're having is what others have told you is what happy is?

Are you happy because the dictionary definition of happy defines your emotions right now?

How about now?

And . . . how about now?

What people who are open about their struggle often do not recognize is that the people who appear to be quite happy are also struggling with something.

Am I struggling right now?

Yes, and I am also happy.

Sometimes, I get hurt and I know this, therefore, I have dedicated myself to my healing.

If someone told you that you cannot both struggle and experience happiness, at the same time; they are not properly informed.

If you really want to be happy you must understand that happiness is an illusion, if you believe it to be.

And . . . Happiness is real if you believe it to be.

And ... Happiness is _____.

Happiness is an Illusion, or is it? WORKSHEET

1.   A simple and difficult question to begin with, simply: are you happy?

2.   What are three things that you do when you don't feel well to feel better?

3.   Based on everything you know about life and about living as yourself; is your happiness a choice?

How to Heal from Betrayal and Find Peace in Your Heart

One of the worst feelings a person can experience is that of being betrayed.

To put your trust in another is a priceless sharing of your soul.

When things go awry, between you and another, it can feel like your heart has been ripped out of your chest, stomped on and set on fire.

We are born trusting of others. Our Parents, Our Teachers, Our Doctors and Our Families.

What do you do when this trust is betrayed?

What do you do when this trust is betrayed when you are a child?

What do you do when the damage is severe?

Maybe if it was tomorrow when I was writing this passage, I would have a better and more well developed answer.

Thankfully, it is today and I don't feel so well, so you get a real and raw answer to the question posed above.

How am I to heal from this betrayal and return the peace to my heart?

This book exists as part of my quest to figure this out.

Please let me know if you figure this out; your input will be quite appreciated.

How to Heal from Betrayal and Find Peace in Your Heart WORKSHEET

1. What is your suggestion to me and the world on how to heal from betrayal and return peace to our hearts? This ain't no joke, I'm asking for your help. Please send me your answer via the contact information on the back cover of this book.

2. If you've been betrayed by those we are naturally expected to be able to trust in this world, what steps have you taken to be able to learn to trust yourself as you live your life's journey forward?

3. I know that if you're reading this, that at one point or another in your life, you considered what the world would be like if you were no longer in it. The fact that you're alive means you love yourself in one way or another. That is solid gold in your spiritual fuel tank. Please ponder this question; why do you get up every day and do whatever you do to be here right now?

Revolution Comes from Within

Paris, France 10:59AM, March 2018

I am surrounded by survivors from a dozen nations.

Everyone is wonderful here. Truly.

This building is home to two dozen broken hearts; all of whom have chosen to live.

A young man who has recently witnessed ultimate horrors, said to me, "we're all brothers here."

He and his brother offered me space to join them, sleeping on a queen-sized mattress; and I did.

People who have experienced their world being demolished, understand the world in ways that not all do.

It is not hard to feel the energy of liberty; in this revolutionary space.

Two dozen broken hearts, united by something there are no words to describe, ain't just c'est bon; c'est magnifique.

Paris, France 11:20AM, March 2018

You are this revolutionary space; you must be your revolution; it must come from within.

Any human who chooses to be this revolution becomes their dreams.

It is the power created when your old life collides with your new life.

Are you facing your end or do you know you are facing your beginning?

There is a magical space that exists between these two realities.

For a beginning to exist there must be an end.

The questions of why are we alive, why are we here and why do we exist; are found in the space between the beginning and the end.

Perhaps most are afraid of tasting something often deemed forbidden?

Perhaps ...

Revolution Comes from Within WORKSHEET

1.   If you feel that some of the questions in these worksheets are repetitive, you are correct. So, let me ask you again, because you matter: what are you doing today to be the best version of yourself possible?

2.   What's the craziest thing you've ever done in your attempt to be happy, to be well, to be successful, to be satisfied and to be the embodiment of whatever it is you were born to be?

3.   Who were you born to be? And if you think that's a hard question, you're correct. Thankfully, that doesn't matter; so, who were you born to be?

How To Manage Public Meltdowns

The Humiliation . . . it will devastate you.

I know the burning sting; do you?

Do they think I am crazy?

How can I ever show my face again?

Am I better off dead?

Does anyone have any idea how terrible I feel?

I must be truly alone.

Does anyone know that my, "Craig had a public meltdown again" is an expression of my deepest raw despair?

To the person reading this; I know the shame that comes from "losing your shit" publicly.

I want you to know that you are not alone and I know you have heard this hundreds of times.

You have heard it from Suicide Prevention Hotlines, your family, your community, your therapist, your peer supporter . . . .

You know when they speak those words, while they may mean what they say with sincerity, even with love; you also know that what they say means nothing . . .

Do my words hurt? Is it because you are hearing or reading someone speak the forbidden truth or is it because you know it is true?

How To Manage Public Meltdowns

1. As evident by you reading this, you clearly survived everything that has ever happened to you. Therefore, curiosity begs the question: of all the crazy shit you've ever done what, can you laugh about?

2. Most people who experience public meltdowns have considered leaving this planet due to the shame and for other reasons; why are you alive today?

3. Do you believe that by having your deepest rawest and most desperate pains understood and validated, that you would experience healing?

And in defiance I still choose love

Stripped me naked publicly

Burned me 1,000 times with 100 cigarettes

Slashed my body with a rusty knife

Beat me between my legs with a metal pipe

Doused my raw body in rubbing alcohol

Beat what's left of me black and blue

Leaving me on the street to die

And in defiance I still choose love.

"Believe in miracles . . .

Because the words you just read are written by one."